How to Lose Weight Well

Easy Steps to Lose Weight by Eating

Table of Contents

quality. Trademarks mentioned are done without written consent and can in no way be considered an endorsement from the trademark holder.

Introduction

Congratulations on purchasing this book and thank you for doing so. This book will discuss the ways in which you can lose weight by eating well. It is a comprehensive guide on eating right to burn excess fat and achieve a healthy body.

Belly bulges aren't pleasant. They not only present a problem for your style quotient but also dent your overall personality. Pounds of flesh bulging out of clothes is a horrific dream for many. It isn't a pleasant imagination even overweight people. Yet, most of the overweight people know they are slowly reaching that stage.

Obesity is a stark reality of this era. It has gripped the modern world firmly. With more than 70% of US population falling in the overweight category and 39.8% in the obese category, the prognosis doesn't look good. The worse part, we know about it. The scary part, on a broader scale, is that the efforts to counter obesity have largely proven to be ineffective.

This is a reality that we all know. We are quite familiar with the harmful effects of obesity. It is a very unpleasant condition.

Obesity is a life-limiting condition. It is much more than simply accumulating some extra pounds of flesh. Other than excess weight issues, obesity brings with itself a lot of other problems too. Hypertension, cardiovascular diseases, metabolic disorders, and other such issues are among them. The extra weight causes extra stress on your joints. It limits your movement, hence, also limits your ability to shed the weight. And yet, we all know these simple facts.

The real quest is for the solution. One bright idea that can help you in getting rid of these extra pounds–a solution that can help you shed the extra weight and also help in sustaining it.

This one quest has led to the unprecedented success of the weight loss industry–an industry which has a market of more than $66 billion today. In a matter of a few decades, from nothing to billions of dollars is quite a leap. It also stresses the fact that obesity has become a very big problem quite recently.

However, the scarier part is that in spite of the steep growth of the weight loss industry, the obesity problem is also growing at the same rate. It is a clear indicator of the ineffectiveness of current measures. It means that something is amiss. There is some important piece in the puzzle that we are missing entirely.

People have gotten so obsessed with the idea of losing weight that they are ready to adopt any measure. From fad diets to killing exercise routines, from obesity pills to weight loss surgeries, people are ready to go to extremes to shed the weight. However, there is a slight problem. The weight comes back and it will keep coming back even after repeated attempts if there is no sustainability.

The biggest reason for the increasing rate of obesity and dissatisfaction among the general public is the ineffectiveness of weight loss measures. Either the weight loss measures do not yield results at all or, even more, the weight comes back after some time of losing it. Strict diets, hard exercise routines, pills, surgeries, meal supplements, and other such measures can help in losing some weight initially but most of these measures are not sustainable in the long run. Hence, weight relapse occurs almost certainly.

All those people who are trying to lose weight through fast but unsustainable methods are likely to get disappointed in the end. A crucial thing that weight loss industry clearly fails to convey is that maintaining a healthy weight and body is a continuous process. Going on some super strict diet for 15 days or 6 months cannot help you in remaining fit. Your excess weight is not an ailment which can be cured through some pill. When you try to shed extra weight or reduce the fat bulges in your body, you are actually trying to go against the natural process of your body. You can neither rush this process nor stop it.

Your body will keep trying to accumulate weight for the whole span of your life. It is in the body's survival instinct. If you want to remain fit and healthy, you will have to work for the whole of your life to keep the weight under control. Anything above and beyond this is cosmetic measure and will not work for long.

The real problem with weight loss measures like fad diets, strict exercise routines, and lengthy meal plans is that people can't follow them for very long. As soon as you get off your calorie restrictive diet, you want to eat. You want to make up for all the food and taste you have lost. This is counterproductive. Even if you follow strict control, your body keeps pushing you.

The same goes for exercise routines. While you are pumping iron in the gym, your food intake increases. You eat more calories because you are burning more. Your appetite increases. However, as soon as you stop working, those extra calories start getting accumulated as fat. You can stop exercise without prior notice, but the same doesn't go with an appetite.

The biggest problem with most weight loss measure is that they propagate food as your biggest enemy. Food is projected as the biggest reason for fat accumulation and therefore every effort is made to limit food intake.

Food is not your enemy but a requirement of life. You cannot lose weight and maintain it too until you accept this fact wholeheartedly. Embracing food as your partner in shedding extra weight and maintaining a healthy body is the best approach.

This book presents a holistic approach to weight loss.

One of the biggest limiting factors in weight loss is not the kind and amount of food items we eat, but also our overall psychology. This book will walk you through those factors and help you in effective weight loss.

Too many fad diets, strict food plans, and tough exercise routines can bring short-term reliefs. However, in the long run, such success stories don't shine much. This book will serve you as a guide to sustainable ways to lose weight by eating right. It is the most effective way to lose weight and maintain it. We cannot expect to remain fit and healthy by having grudges about food. The best way to have a healthy body is to embrace the food that we eat. You will be able to identify the right food items and the benefits they bring.

One of the biggest factors that lead to excess weight is craving for food. Although eating is natural to any living being, craving is not. It is a result of bad eating habits and poor food choices.

✓ This book will explain the natural ways to avoid craving and overeating.
✓ It will explain the benefits of natural foods for weight loss and help you in creating a natural food plan.
✓ In this book, you'll also get ample of breakfast, lunch, and dinner ideas to keep you healthy and fit.
✓ You'll also get to know about healthy fruits to add to your meal for best results.
✓ A healthy weight loss plan is the one which leads to faster fat burn and slows muscle loss. This book will give you exactly the same.
✓ You can get all that without crushing diets and unhealthy food regimen.

Simply read the book and embrace the idea of healthy living by eating well.
There are plenty of books on this subject on the market, thanks again for choosing this one! Every effort was made to

ensure it is full of as much useful information as possible. Please enjoy!

BONUS:

As a way of saying thank you for purchasing my book, please use your link below to claim your 3 FREE Cookbooks on Health, Fitness & Dieting Instantly

https://bit.ly/2EFv31x

You can also share your link with your friends and families whom you think that can benefit from the cookbooks or you can forward them the link as a gift!

Chapter 1: Understanding Weight Loss Psychology

Weight loss is an important goal. Health is and should be of paramount importance for all. If your health starts failing you, then enjoying other pleasures of life becomes difficult. One of the biggest hurdles in the way of achieving good health is excess weight.

Excess weight not only affects your personality and performance but also affects your psychology and attitude. However, most of us look at it in the wrong way. Most people try to make their excess weight a scapegoat for all that has gone wrong in their life.

It is easy to blame things that are not going to answer you back. But, if you look closely, you'll find that excess weight does not necessarily bring bad things into your life. It is usually the other way around and weight accumulation is a consequence of wrong lifestyle habits. So, if you start improving things in life, weight issues can be countered with greater ease.

In the hurry to lose weight, we tend to overlook the factors that lead to weight gain in the first place. We will need to admit and understand the fact that the human brain functions in a very sophisticated way. The first priority of the brain is to keep you alive in all situations. It looks at things from a very different perspective. Your body is a coordinated machine that takes every step to ensure survival. Therefore, it starts hoarding energy if it senses any kind of stress or danger. Hence, ignoring even the small things can have a huge impact on your weight.

If you want to lose weight, then it is important that you understand the factors that affect your weight. Ignoring these factors will lead to failures and disappointments.

Stress

Living the life of a sage is not an option these days. It is the age of competition. It always has been so as the whole theory of evolution is based on the principle of 'survival of the fittest'. Yet, the competition has attained a whole new dimension in the modern world. You need to excel in school as well as your workplace. You need to be better than your peers and work harder. Achieve deadlines and perform harder. However, this fierce competition takes away your focus from health and gives way to stress. Both the things are bad for you.

Stress is not good for you. It not only affects your heart and brain but it also affects your weight in many ways. When you are stressed, your body starts releasing a stress hormone called 'cortisol'. This hormone causes various problems, but the biggest one is that it signals your body to increase the storage of fat. So, if you are living a stressful life, then this hormone will sabotage all your efforts to lose weight.

People leading a stressful life also find great solace in food as it is distracting and relieving. Stressful situations invoke a fight-or-flight response. This elevates the need to consume more calories. People end up eating sugary and fatty foods in such circumstances. They all lead to excess calorie intake that is completely unnecessary. Your body is already in low-fat burning mode due to high cortisol release; therefore, all those calories end up getting stored as fat. Sweets and processed fatty foods which you like so much in such situations are addictive and you tend to develop a taste and craving for them pretty soon. This leads to quicker weight gain.

In this age of competition, it would be impractical to advise leading a completely stress-free life. However, trying to reduce stress is a very practical and doable thing. If you really want your weight loss efforts to work and get fit, then start trying to handle the stress wisely. It is a daemon that will cause more damage than you can think.

There are several ways to lower your stress levels. Enjoying your time with friends and family, meditation, light exercise, and indulging in recreational activities can help you in lowering your stress levels to a great extent. You will not only feel better but will also lose weight much faster. Remember, losing weight isn't simply adjusting your calorie intake. Your body has the ability to decrease or increase the metabolism as per its need. If you are leading a stressful life, then eating a lower number of calories also may not help you much in shedding weight. Your body will start conserving every bit of it. The more relaxed you are, the better your metabolism will be.

Pleasure

It is simply the opposite phenomenon of stress. It relaxes you and your body too. If you are in a pleasant mood, you respond to situations in a better way in real life. In the same way, pleasure relaxes your body too. Cortisol release reduces and your body comes out of the survival mode. It can safely increase the metabolic rate, as it senses no danger for conserving energy. Your gut starts functioning better and digests food easily.

The first step towards achieving a healthy body is to relax. At least while you are eating, take off your mind from stressful things. Give your mind the time to enjoy the food. The more you feel, smell, and enjoy the food the better your body will be able to process it effectively.

If you enjoy the aroma of the food before eating it, your digestive system goes into an overdrive. It will start pumping the digestive juices and you will be able to digest the food quickly. Taking a moment to enjoy the foods leads to fulfillment quite fast. You will not have frequent cravings for food.

Mindset

Food gives you energy. If you eat an excess of it, then it will lead to excess weight. It is not the food that leads to weight gain your negligent behavior towards it. It is very important that you start looking at food with a positive approach.

Eating the right kind of things in the right proportions will make you healthy and will also help you in losing weight.

Some people outrightly reject certain kinds of foods and heavily advocate others. This is an approach that can be harmful. Ultimately, it is not the food that is causing weight gain but its excessive consumption. All foods have one or the other nutrient and you need all of them in certain proportions. The important thing is to understand those proportions and to stick to them.

You will have to accept the fact that you cannot lose weight by simply avoiding food, as most diets suggest. This strategy doesn't work for long. Living on a calorie-restrictive diet for the whole life is not only challenging but also impractical.

You will have to develop a mindset where you acknowledge the benefits of food items and consume them in a proportionate manner. This will help you in losing weight and maintaining it easily.

People want to lose weight but do not get the right way to do so and so they look for it in all directions. The flourishing weight loss industry is a bright example of the same.

You cannot become healthy by avoiding food or adopting superficial methods to burn fat. You cannot remain on calorie restrictive diets forever. Pumping iron in the gym on a regular basis is also not an option for most people, as they have to tend to other important needs of life and family. The best option in front of you in such circumstances is to make food your partner in losing weight.

Healthy food choices and good eating habits can help you in enjoying your life while keeping it tasty. The weight loss industry has created a myth that weight loss is a tough process which can only be achieved by eating tasteless food and sacrificing your pleasures of taste. Their whole idea makes weight loss look like a very tough activity.

If you want to lose weight then you will have to understand the psychology of weight loss. If you are too stressed about your weight, then your weight loss process will slow down. The more stress-free you remain, the faster you'll lose weight. You will have to become more accepting of the power of food. It can help you in losing weight without much noise. You simply need to select the right food to eat and follow a healthy lifestyle. The more natural these things remain, the more sustainable your weight loss will be.

Motivation

Motivation is the fuel for success. The right motivation keeps you going irrespective of the challenges. The biggest problem in weight loss comes in the form of correcting some poor lifestyle habits. If you do not have the right motivation, you can easily give in to the temptation and your whole weight loss attempt would go for a toss. If you have a strong motivation behind losing weight, you'll be able to win over temptations easily. Find a strong motivation to lose weight and keep working towards it at a steady pace.

You can easily lose weight if you make healthy food choices and adopt good eating habits. The following chapter will put forward some important food tips that can help you in losing weight easily.

Chapter 2: Key Points to Consider for Healthy Eating

Most people believe they can control weight by simply regulating the number of calories they take. This is a wrong notion. Although it is a fact that extra calories do add fat but all calories are not the same. Different food items have much more than simple calories. If you want to lose weight through eating well, then you will have to switch to healthy eating habits.

Healthy eating means adding the right foods that give you the required nutrients. Eating foods that give you empty calories will simply add to the weight. Food items that spike insulin levels will not help your weight loss either. Therefore, it is important that you adopt some good eating habits for faster results.

Focus on Fiber

Fiber is the key to weight loss. It is one food ingredient that can help you lose weight in many ways.

The fiber in fruits, vegetables, and whole foods is slow to digest. It is good for your gut and fills up your stomach fast and keeps it occupied for long. This helps in avoiding cravings for food and improves your digestive system. Apart from that, fiber-rich vegetables are low on calories and therefore you have no danger of adding extra weight by eating fiber. Green leafy vegetables have lots of fiber and mineral but negligible calories. You can eat them as much as you want without worrying about weight.

Apart from fruits and vegetables, whole grains are also a rich source of fiber. Dietary fiber is not only good for your digestion system but it also helps in keeping your insulin levels under check.

Have a Crush on Whole Foods

Whole grains are great. They are a rich source of carbohydrates. Although carbohydrates are advertised as a no-go by most health experts, whole grains are good. Apart from carbohydrates, whole grains also provide a lot of dietary fiber, as well as trace nutrients like vitamins and minerals. These are very important for your well being and there are many nutrients that you don't from other sources.

The dietary fiber in whole grains keeps your digestive system healthy and engaged. It will not only decrease your weight but also the risk of serious problems like hypertension, heart diseases, and digestive problems.

Healthy Fat is Important

The weight loss industry has demonized fat and cholesterol as the root cause of all evil. This is wrong. Fat is very important. In fact, your body cannot function properly without fat and cholesterol. Fat and cholesterol are building blocks of the hormones in your body. It won't function without fat. Fat provides long-lasting sustainable energy to your body.

However, as all fat is not bad, most kinds of fats are not good either. Bad quality of fat consumed by eating fried foods, sauces, and hydrogenated oils is very unhealthy. It will increase your weight and speed up the process of clogging your arteries.

To remain healthy, you need to consume healthy fats. Fatty fish, nuts, olive oil, avocados, and other such things provide you the required healthy fats. You need to embrace them to remain healthy and fit.

Don't Miss Out on Protein

Protein is the building block of muscles. When you start losing weight, you don't simply lose fat, but also lose a lot of muscle mass. This can cause problems if you are not eating protein in the right quantity.

Eating a high protein diet also has an added advantage; it makes you feel full faster. A protein rich diet means that you will achieve satiety sooner and will not have food cravings. However, you must remember the fact that protein also has calories and so you must tread the path carefully.

Avoid Refined Sugar at All Costs

Added sugar in all forms is bad for your health. Refined sugar not only spikes your insulin levels but it also dumps a lot of empty calories, both of which are bad. If you want to lose weight fast and maintain a healthy lifestyle, then cutting on the refined sugar should be your first step. If you have a sweet tooth, then look for natural sweeteners like fruits. They are sweet but contain fructose which is healthy.

Refined sugar is addictive. The more you eat it, the more you would want very soon. This means that you will never have enough of it. Your weight loss plans will go down the drain. The best way to avoid temptation is to stay completely away from them. Even a small amount of refined sugar will keep causing problems for you.

One big hurdle in staying away from refined sugar is processed foods. They have high quantities of refined sugar to add taste. This makes them unhealthy and avoidable. If you want to lose weight, you will also have to cut down your processed food intake.

Stay Away from Easy Calories

Simplifying your food may not be the best solution for you all the time. When your body takes time in digesting something, it burns calories in the process. Your metabolism goes up and the process of losing weight gets in place. Therefore, it is best to eat food items as close to their natural state as possible. Although this doesn't mean that you need to eat whole foods raw or vegetables uncooked, still try to follow it as closely as possible.

When you eat a fruit in the natural state, it takes time to get digested. The release of calories is slow and your digestive system remains engaged in sending a signal of satiety. However, if you drink the juice of the same fruit, the calorie influx is high and sudden, but short-lived. You'll feel hungry soon and will consume more but unnecessary calories.

The same goes for all kinds of health drinks, carbonated beverages, and the likes. They all add extra calories to your body without providing anything to your digestive system. Your insulin levels remain spiked and the added sugar in these drinks leads to cravings.

It doesn't matter what the label of the energy drink says. If it has any kind of taste or flavor, it isn't natural and should be avoided. All energy drinks and zero-calorie drinks carry this risk. If you are thirsty and dehydrated, drink water and nothing else.

Do not try to simplify your food. Eating food as close to their natural state as possible is the best way to lose weight. The longer your digestive system takes to process it, the better.

Refined Carbs are Bad

Empty calories in all forms are bad and refined carbs just bring that to you. Refined carbs lack the essential fiber and nutrients and load you with calories. They are bad for your digestive system and spike your insulin levels.

They raise too many red flags as far as your health is concerned and therefore, you must avoid refined carbs as much as possible.

Mindful Eating is the Key

One of the biggest reasons for binge eating is mindless eating. It is not the taste, smell, hunger, or craving that leads to excess eating; it is simply being mindless about the disadvantages of eating more. When you pay less attention to the food and the quantity you are eating, all the advantages go down the drain.

Eating is an important activity. It is essential for your survival. Eating while watching TV, or talking can take away your mind from it and it leads to overeating. You would want to avoid that if you are trying to lose weight.

Always watch the things you are eating and be cautious about the quantity.

Chapter 3: How to Stop Dieting and Other Strict Food Plans

The plain and simple fact is that diets and strict food plans are short-term weight loss strategies and they don't work out in the long run. Diets are restrictive and anything that's restrictive works against human nature. As soon as people get off diet plans they start gaining weight. Even if they remain on a diet plan for a bit longer, the results start to go down. Watching your labor go down the drain can be frustrating.

However, some people still like to follow diets and strict food plans as it gives them a sense of control. They feel that they are steering their life in the direction they want. But, this feeling soon turns counterproductive when they hit a plateau. This not only adds to the exasperation but also leads to stress. Some people still like to stick to diets as they feel they'll become vulnerable once they get off the diet. It is a negative feeling.

Food is an important part of life and picturing it as a villain is not going to work. You will have to get off the diet plans if you want to lose weight and maintain it successfully.

Diets and restrictive food plans are devised to work against the human constitution. Our body goes into the survival mode as soon as we lower our calorie intake. It reduces the metabolic rate and our body adjusts to the low-calorie intake. So, although the diets may seem to work in the beginning, they become ineffective over a period.

If you take a short-term diet plan, you may feel a bit of weight loss. Generally, it is the water weight that goes down but it bounces back very fast. People on a diet tend to indulge in binge eating due to natural instincts which also leads to excess weight gain very fast.

The best way to lose weight and maintain it for a long period is to stop dieting or following other strict food plans. Eating well and following a healthy eating regimen will help you much effectively in losing weight.

So, even if you have indulged in binge eating after getting off a diet, the best thing to do is not to get on another diet plan. You may feel tempted to do so but it is a bad move. Food is a requirement of life and our body can process it. You can work out a bit more and handle those extra calories. Your fat metabolism will be better if you stop stressing about some extra calories. Stress is bad for fat-burning. So, embrace the fact that you have eaten some extra calories and move on.

When you aren't on a diet you are free to eat anything, as there is no restriction. This will make food items less seductive or appealing to you. This is the first step to success. You can choose to eat or not eat anything without guilt. This works better than any diet for your body.

People who have been following diet plans for long may find it difficult, but it is the fact. Getting on a diet is not going to fetch results. You will only get results when you follow a healthy eating routine.

Technical Problems with Diet Plans

Most diet plans focus on one part of the problem and that is high-calorie intake. They work on reducing the calorie intake. However, that isn't the best thing to do. Whatever we eat adds calories to our body. Those calories help us in running the body and the extra ones pile up as fat. But, all calories are not equal. For instance, let us consider the macronutrients.

❖ **Carbohydrate**

Carbohydrate is the main energy fuel. The more carbohydrate we eat the easier our calorie procurement gets. Lowering the carbohydrate intake will make energy production tough. So, lowering carbohydrate intake judiciously is a wise step.

❖ **Protein**

Protein intake also adds calories but has a very different function. Protein is needed for muscle building. If you lower your protein intake on a diet then you will face problems in muscle building. If you lower your carbohydrate intake too much, your body will start eating up your muscles for energy. That's why a very strict diet will lead to muscle loss. Proteins need to be part of your meal in a balanced manner.

❖ **Fat**

Fat is another important macronutrient. It plays several important functions in your body. All the hormones are made from cholesterol and it is a product of fat. Therefore, your body cannot survive without the fat intake. Reducing the fat intake can prove to be detrimental to your health. High fat and cholesterol levels can spell problems for you but it doesn't come from your healthy fats. Dietary cholesterol is safe. If you remove healthy fats from your diet it is going to be bad for your health.

The real problem with diets is that they generally cut out on all these macronutrients and therefore end up ruining your health.

The weight loss industry and food product manufacturing companies have projected fat as the real devil. It has been established in common perception that if you eat fat, you'll get fat. It is an absurd idea. Mankind has been surviving on fat for thousands of years. Fat has been the main food source for human beings since the beginning and we had even made it through the dark ages. One thing that has got added very recently is the main cause of the obesity problem and that's *Refined SUGAR*. Mankind had no access to refined sugar for centuries. It is a recent addition to our food. In fact, the trend of processed food is also very recent and major cause of the problem. High dependence on processed foods has brought a lot of refined sugar in our lives and we have gotten fatter since.

Diets try to target the problem in a wrong way. You can lower your calorie intake but can't force your body to burn its fat deposits, not until it has the right signals from the brain. The main hormone responsible for fat storage is insulin. Until there is insulin present in your bloodstream your body will not start burning fat deposits. Insulin keeps sending a signal to your fat cells that there is an abundance of food and they need to store fat. If you want to burn fat, then you will have to devise ways to ensure that your insulin release gets regulated. Carbohydrates spike up your insulin levels easily. Refined sugar seriously messes up with insulin levels. But, fat doesn't lead to insulin release. Therefore, fat diet is not the problem; low-fat diet is the real culprit as it has a lot of added sugar in it. If you want to lower your weight, you will have to regulate your insulin levels and carbohydrate intake. Lowering fat and protein intake will only cause problems.

Diets and strict food plans also create a craving for food in you. Such plans cannot be followed for long and when you get off such plans, you start gaining weight fast. The best way to avoid such situations is to stop following diets and start following a healthy eating routine.

The first step towards a healthy diet is to minimize the consumption of processed food. Your focus should not be simply to minimize the consumption of calories but to eat the right things. It is only through eating well that you can lose weight.

It is important to make it clear in your mind that your body has evolved through centuries. It has a very sophisticated system designed to prolong survival. If you are planning to reduce the weight by survival then you are heading on a road to failure and the journey is bounding to be painful. As you lower the calorie intake, the body will lower the metabolism to ensure lower energy consumption. This gives it more time to survive. Mankind hasn't survived through floods, droughts, and famines without merit.

If you want to pin down your weight, then you will have to hit the fat in the right way. Triggering the hormones that help in fat burning is the best way to ensure weight loss. Your body will only start burning fat stores when it is sure that it isn't in danger or there is no dearth of energy supply.

Insulin is the key hormone that blocks any kind of fat burning. If you want to lose weight then you will have to regulate insulin levels in your body. Shortage or excess of food will only cause erratic insulin levels and that must be avoided at all costs.

The main function of insulin is to facilitate blood glucose absorption. Foods that take time to get digested and do not cause sudden insulin spikes are the best.

Refined sugar stands at the top of the list of foods that must be avoided. If you like eating sweets or processed food items, then your insulin levels are bound to be erratic. Fiber-rich foods are the best when it comes to normalizing your insulin levels. They take time to get digested and do not cause sudden insulin spikes.

Choosing healthy food items rich in fiber, minerals, and vitamins will help you a lot. Green leafy vegetables stand out on the list, as they are rich in mineral and fiber and add a negligible amount of calories.

People generally adopt diet routines as they are unhappy with their bodies and want to regain control. However, diets can cause stress and anxiety due to slow progress. They also lead to fear of failure which is not good either for your physique or for your mind. Diets restrict you and lead to food cravings that can be emotionally taxing. Eating anything not on the list can also give way to guilty consciousness. Losing weight on such terms is unhealthy. There is bound to be a rebound even if you lose some weight through such measures.

The best way to get off diets is to understand that you can only lose weight in a sustainable manner if you follow a healthy routine, a routine that can last long and doesn't cause so much mental and emotional anxiety. Avoiding food is not the solution but a problem.

If you eat on a healthy, balanced diet, you can easily lose weight.

The first thing to do is avoid the intake of refined sugar. This means that processed food items should be consumed with great caution. The more you eat natural food products the better it will be for your weight loss goals.

The refined sugar is addictive and creates a craving for food. This leads to piling up of empty calories that do nothing besides spiking your insulin levels. You must avoid such foods.

Carbonated drinks, sodas, energy drinks, and alcohol have high quantities of sugar. You must avoid them as much as possible. They will not only spike your blood sugar levels but also make you crave for more very often.

Avoiding low-fat food is also a good idea. Low-fat foods have lots of added sugar in them as without fat the food starts tasting bad. To compensate for the loss of taste food product, manufacturers load them with added sugar. This is a strong reason to ditch low-fat food. You should stick to natural fruits, vegetables, and whole grains; they will provide you all the required macronutrient and help in regulating insulin levels.

Insulin is the key to weight loss. It is the key to health. You will have to adopt food items that help you in keeping your insulin levels in check.

Mindfulness in eating will help you a lot in weight loss. Your aim should be to consume the required amounts of calories with a good balance of all the macronutrients. Simply cutting down the calories wouldn't work. Cutting down of calories means cutting down on protein as well as fats. This can be unhealthy. You don't only want to lose weight but be fit and healthy too. An unhealthy diet cannot make you healthy.

The best way to beat the weight is to remain happy and content. The more accepting you are towards food the less problematic it will be for you.

Chapter 4: Learn the Ways to Suppress Cravings and Overeating Sprees

Craving for food is one of the biggest enemies of weight loss measures. Your craving for food can compel you to eat unhealthy things that just lead to weight gain. It is a compelling feeling that leads to guilt and stress later on.

Learning to tackle the strong urge to eat or cravings is an important thing. Craving for food doesn't arise out of thin air. Some people take it upon themselves that they cannot control their cravings. There is no need to be so hard upon yourself. Cravings are as much a physiological phenomenon as they are emotional.

When you haven't eaten for some time, you start feeling hungry, it is a normal thing. But, there are times when you aren't even particularly hungry but want to eat something. There may be times when you have eaten your fill but you want to keep eating more. This is craving.

Craving for more food can arise out of your inflated energy needs. However, if that's the case, you'll know and there is no reason to worry. But, if your energy needs are the same and you still feel frequent cravings for food then there can be several reasons for that which you need to understand.

Some Important Causes of Unexplained Cravings

Wrong Food Items

Almost always, the cravings are for sweets and processed foods. Junk foods and processed foods contain lots of added sugar. This sugar is addictive and makes you long for more. The more you will eat them, the more you'll want to eat them. They'll keep dragging you down. There is no way of getting around them. Controlling your refined sugar intake is the best way to suppress cravings. If you frequently long for sweets, you should switch to fruits. Fruits contain fructose which can easily be processed by your body. Besides fructose, fruits also contain a lot of fiber. You'll feel satisfied after eating comparatively small amounts of fruits. This will help you in fighting your cravings for sweets.

Processed and fast foods can make you long for more. They contain a lot of empty calories. The high amount of added sugar makes these foods tasty and you want to eat more. These are unhealthy foods and besides calories, you also get lots of bad cholesterol from these foods. Avoiding them is the best way to suppress the cravings. The longer you stay away from such foods, the fewer cravings you will have for them.

Hormonal Imbalance

Leptin is an important hormone in your body that induces satiety. It sends signals to your brain that you have eaten enough and you don't need to eat more. However, inflammation in the fat cells can lead to unregulated leptin release. This phenomenon can trigger leptin resistance and you may have cravings for food even after eating. Eating healthy anti-inflammatory foods and maintaining a healthy lifestyle can help you in dealing with this problem.

Stress

Stress is a leading cause of food craving. Some people try to find solace in food when they find themselves in stressful situations. Others wrongly treat food to be a solution for their depression. This is wrong and getting out of it is very important. Ignoring such cravings can lead to serious weight gain. Food cannot be a solution to your emotional problems. On the contrary, it will aggravate the emotional issues in more ways than one. Getting help from the expert is the best way to get out of stress as food can't be the solution.

Choosing healthy food items over junk foods is the best way to deal with cravings. If you are having cravings for specific food items, then try to replace them with similar but healthy things.

Some items that most people crave for are:

1. Chocolates: Chocolate tops the list when it comes to food items that cause cravings. Magnesium deficiency in your body can lead to cravings for chocolate as it is rich in it. However, there are many other healthy foods that are rich in magnesium like avocados and almonds. You should opt for them in place of chocolate when you feel the urge.

2. Potato Chips: Craving for potato chips can be pretty strong but it is very unhealthy. It is highly processed and adds too much salt to your body. You can eat nuts in place of chips. They not only contain healthy fats but also make you feel fuller fast.

3. Pastries and Candies: These have lots of refined sugar and are very bad for you. They'll make you long for more. The best way to avoid the cravings for these is to replace them with fruits like peaches, cherries, or melons. Dried fruits like prunes or raisins are also a very good replacement for candies and pastries.

4. Soda and other sweetened beverages: Soda and other such drinks are bad for your health. They are addictive and make you long for more. They supply a lot of unnecessary calories even if they are advertised as zero-calorie drinks. The best way to deal with the cravings for such beverages is to replace them with fresh lime water or unsweetened tea or coffee.

Best Way to Reduce Craving and Overeating

Drink Plenty of Water

If you crave for something, drinking water will help you a lot. Water makes you feel fuller and subsides the craving. It is a calorie-free drink and hydrates you. You can drink water without the fear of loading yourself with extra calories. Drinking plenty of water not only lowers your appetite but also helps in weight loss. So, you'll be killing two birds with one stone by drinking plenty of water when you feel a craving for food. First, you will suppress your hunger and second, you'll increase your resting energy expenditure. This consumes calories and helps in faster weight loss.

Eat Protein Rich Diet

High protein diet is known to reduce your craving for food significantly. It makes you feel full for longer and you do not feel the craving for food. Eating a protein-rich diet also helps you in muscle building which is important while you are trying to lose weight as loss of muscle mass is higher during weight loss.

Create Distraction

Food can be tempting especially the one you crave for. The best way to avoid cravings is to stay away from such foods. If you feel tempted to eat something then creating a distraction is the best way to stop yourself from eating it. Going on a brisk walk or engaging in some other physical activity is a good way to avoid such cravings. Chewing gums or eating low-calorie foods like vegetables can also help you in curbing the urge.

Plan Your Meals in Advance

Planning is the key to healthy living. If you want to make healthy food choices then planning in advance is the best. This way, you'll stay away from the temptation of going for fast food or processed meals. Such foods will only create a craving for more and dump empty calories in your system. If possible, plan your meals in advance. Prepare healthy meals and load your fridge with fruits and vegetables. In this way, you can avoid the temptation of taking the shortcuts like fast food. Planned food is nutritious and helps in suppressing the urge to eat more.

Avoid Staying Hungry for Long

You should maintain healthy breaks between meals but never starve yourself for long. When you stay away for long, your body starts looking for quick energy. Eating at planned intervals keeps you full and you can avoid cravings and hunger pangs easily. Ultimately, you stay fuller and eat healthily.

Avoid Stress

Stress can cause strong cravings. Additionally, when you are stressed your body starts releasing cortisol which can lead to weight gain. Under stress, people resort to binge eating and give in to cravings. The best way to deal with this problem is to avoid stress. Engage in healthy activities like socializing with friends and family and doing some outdoor games or other recreational activities. This lowers your stress hormones and your cravings for food go down.

Mindful Eating is the Key

Most of us do not pay much attention to our food. It is an important part of our lives and needs our due attention. Mindful eating helps us in eating in a controlled manner. We also understand the positives and negatives of the food we eat and can easily avoid unhealthy foods. It is the best way to avoid impulsive eating. While you are eating stay away from the TV or your smartphone. Do not eat while you are working on your laptop or talking to someone as you will not be able to judge the amount of food you eat. When you are eating mindfully, you are able to judge satiety better.

Eat Slowly

When you are hungry, your gut releases the ghrelin hormone. This hormone signals your brain to induce hunger. As you eat, the ghrelin levels go down and leptin levels increase. The leptin hormone signals your brain that you are feeling satisfied. However, if you eat very fast, your leptin levels will not be able to signal your brain properly. The chances of overeating increase in such circumstances. Eating slow gives your body ample time to sense satiety and you can easily avoid overeating.

Do not keep eating until you start feeling stuffed. The leptin hormone may take some time to completely signal your brain that you are full. Stop eating when you feel a bit full as after some time you will start feeling completely full. Your body needs some time to process the complete amount of food you have eaten and therefore the signals are a bit late.

Sleep is Important

Sleep deprivation can create a strong urge to eat. Proper sleep is important not only for your body but also for your appetite sensors. If you are getting a good sleep, you will feel less hungry and will be able to manage your meals in a healthy manner. Good sleep also helps in proper weight loss as Human Growth Hormone (HGH) release is strongest when you are sleeping. It is one of the most powerful hormones for fat burning. You can burn more fat by sleeping than you can imagine.

Eat Healthy Meals

Meals stacked with empty calories will not only leave you longing for more but will also pile up weight. A balanced meal with all the macronutrients will help you in maintaining a healthy body and staying away from temptations. Your meals must have a healthy balance of good carbohydrates, protein, and healthy fats. Such meals will help you in staying satisfied for long. Pack in as much dietary fiber in your meals as possible. Fiber aids your digestion and keeps your stomach full for long. Whole grains and vegetables are a good source of dietary fiber. If you love fruits, try to eat them in the natural state in place of juicing them. Whole fruits have a lot of fiber which is good for you.

Eat Before You Go Out

You can practically have no control over the food items that you get outside. Going out on an empty stomach is a bad idea as you will be tempted to eat. In this way, you will end up eating unhealthy things and have cravings for more. If you want to avoid such temptations, then always eat before you leave home. Even if you are going for grocery shopping, never go on an empty stomach. An empty stomach will tempt you to buy things that are unhealthy for you. You'll make much wiser food choices when you don't feel tempted to eat anything immediately.

Weight loss is a long-term process. It isn't something that can happen overnight. Even if you achieve significant weight loss quickly, sustaining that success will be very difficult. Making healthy food choices, avoiding cravings, and overeating are the best ways to lose weight and maintain it successfully.

It is a process that will need time, patience, and training. However, it is a very sustainable process as nothing is off-limits for you. You can eat anything you desire once in a while. This freedom liberates you completely and you become less susceptible to give in to seductive foods. This also helps you in engaging in binge eating.

All you need to do is have a bit of patience and start looking at your food more closely. Do not see the food as your foe but consider it a partner in your weight loss. This viewpoint will help you a lot in suppressing the cravings for certain foods.

Chapter 5: Cutting Down Sugar Intake - Most Important Step Towards Weight Loss

When it comes to weight loss nothing can be more detrimental than added sugar. In fact, refined sugar is the most common cause of diseases in our body. It leads to obesity and all other related problems like diabetes, fatty liver, and hypertension.

An average American person consumes more than 145 pounds of added sugar every year. This is without taking into account the amount of hidden sugar you consume through bread, cookies, cereals, crackers, wines, beverages, and processed foods.

Refined sugar spikes your insulin levels. This is one hormone you don't want in high quantities floating in your blood if you are serious about weight loss. Insulin inhibits the release of fat cutting hormones. Several fat-burning hormones like adrenaline and HGH cannot be produced if you have free-flowing insulin in your blood.

If your bloodstream has a high amount of insulin, then your fat stores will focus only on fat storage. The main work of insulin is to help your body cells in the absorption of glucose. Once the need for readily available glucose in the bloodstream is over, the insulin starts storing extra energy in form of glycogen and then as fat. High release of insulin can also lead to insulin resistance. This is a state in which your cells stop responding readily to insulin and your pancreas have to pump out more and more insulin. This insulin resistance even leads to Type 2 Diabetes.

Your belly fat keeps increasing and you gain more weight if the insulin levels remain high. The most common reason for such insulin spikes is sugar.

Refined sugar is a great problem as your body cannot process it directly. The sugar present in fruits is fructose and your body can process it easily. Milk and milk products contain sugar in the form of lactose and your body can process this too. But, the refined sugar is sucrose and your body cannot process it easily. It leads to a sudden spike in energy levels and pumps a lot of empty calories.

The best way to lose weight is to remove refined or added sugar from your daily diet. Although it is a difficult thing if you rely too much on processed food but then losing weight will also become very difficult for you. If you switch to whole foods and natural foods, reducing sugar dependency will become easy.

Some Effective Ways to Cut Sugar Intake

Read the Labels Carefully

Avoiding processed foods completely can be a very tough choice and impractical for many. However, you can still try to avoid sugar as much as possible. While buying anything, read the labels carefully, and look for the amount of sugar present in that food item. The ingredients are listed in the order of their quantity. If the sugar is listed in the top order, that item is best to be avoided. Sugar can be listed by various names like added sugar, natural sugar, syrup, fructose, and other such names. Do not get misguided and look closely. If it is in the middle order or in the lower ranks then that food item would be safer to consume.

Include More Whole Foods in Your Diet

Whole foods like fruits, vegetables, and whole grains contain natural sugar and are very healthy. If you include whole foods in your diet, your dependency or craving for added sugar will go down. Whole foods also contain lots of fiber along with sugar which helps in digestion and keeps you feeling fuller for longer.

Avoid Sweetened Beverages

Sweetened beverages pump a lot of sugar into your system. You'd never even realize the amount of sugar you can consume simply by drinking two cans of soda. Alcohol will load a lot of sugar into your system. Even sweetened coffee or tea has lots of sugar in it. The energy or health drink you drink freely also has lots of refined sugar in it. It is easy to drink a lot of sugar without suspecting. The best way to avoid it is to drink unsweetened beverages. Unsweetened fresh lime or black tea and coffee without sugar are great if you want to drink something.

Don't Get Carried Away by the Tag of Natural Sweeteners

You will never be able to get away from the sugar craving until the time you learn to cut off sugar from your daily diet. Natural sweeteners are simply an excuse and should be avoided. The first few days are tough and you will feel a strong urge to eat sugar but as time passes by you'll feel less inclined to eat sugar. People who simply believe that switching to things carrying natural sweeteners is a better option end up eating more sugar than required. Avoiding it as much as possible is the safest option. Eat fresh fruits if you feel the urge.

Increase Your Protein Intake

Protein in the diet is very satisfying and healthy. It helps you in feeling full for long and guides you in battling with cravings. A protein-rich diet lasts for long so you do not feel the sugar cravings easily. If you feel the need to eat something in between munching on some nuts is a better option than searching for candies and chocolate bars.

Increase Healthy Fats in Your Diet

Food products containing healthy fats are great. They keep you full and do not spike insulin levels. While going for healthy fats, ensure that you rely more on whole foods than simply on oils. Whole foods will give you fiber and other nutrients along with fats and help you all along. A fat rich diet also helps you in curbing the cravings for sweets.

Avoid Temptation

The best way to accidentally bumping into sugary foods is to keep them out of sight at least in your home. If you have chocolates and candies at home, the chances are that you will eat them in weak moments. The best way is to get rid of them. The less you see them, the less inclined you'll feel to eat them.

Do Not Use Sugar as Your Escape Pad

Sugary foods tend to make people feel relaxed. Therefore, people develop a tendency to eat sweets in order to lower their stress level. This is a superficial way to counter stress. If stress is a problem for you, then engage in more reliable pursuits like exercise, games, and other pleasurable activities. Added sugar will remain a worry if you do not handle it is time. The best way to lose weight is a healthy manner is to learn to ditch sugar for good.

Chapter 6: Adopt Natural Foods for Easy Weight Loss

We may not be the oldest or the most primitive species on this earth, yet, we have survived a pretty large amount of time through thick and thin. The human race has survived through 'the Black Plague', floods and famines, deadly diseases, and ages of no cure. We have suffered a large number of problems related to survival through which we sailed, but obesity was never among them. Yet, today in this modern world, aided with all the medical advancement, we are facing an obesity epidemic and struggling to find our way out.

At present, 1.6 billion all over the globe are either obese or overweight and that's from a population of 7 billion. It is the staggering one-fourth of the human race affected by weight issues. Never in history has the complete human race has been affected by one such problem ever. We all know this and in spite of all the modern medical resources at our disposal, we are able to do nothing.

Is it simply a matter of coincidence that humanity has started facing the problem of obesity now? In all likeliness, it cannot be a coincidence. Obesity is a direct result of our poor food choices, overdependence on processed food, and unhealthy lifestyle habits. Therefore, the solution also lies in correcting the same.

The biggest reason behind the obesity epidemic has been an overdependence on processed food. Earlier, our food was basic and simple. We ate food as close to its natural form as possible. It was unadulterated and unprocessed. Today, we eat highly processed food adulterated with artificial sweeteners and fats. This is making us fat and sick. The solution to the problem lies in correcting our food choices and going back to natural foods.

Natural foods can help us in keeping our weight in check and reducing it. We have been consuming them safely for thousands of years without obesity issues. Natural foods are packed with several benefits that help us in staying fit.

Some of the Benefits of Consuming Natural Foods

Packed with Nutrition

Natural foods are packed with nutrition and can help us with weight loss. Food, in its natural form, comes loaded with macronutrients as well as micronutrients. Processing the food erodes the micronutrients in the food. Without proper micronutrients, the food loses its health benefits. A low micronutrient food is less fulfilling and thus leads to overeating. Eating natural foods like whole fruits, vegetables, and whole grains can help you in getting the micronutrients as well as the trace material.

Intact Protein Content

Highly processed food loses its protein content. Either the protein content gets eroded in the processing or becomes very difficult to digest. Several studies have shown that food processing makes several essential amino acids like lysine, tryptophan, methionine, and cysteine less available to the body. The sugar and fats in processed food react with protein and make it complex for human digestion. On the other hand, natural protein-rich food is high in protein and low in calories, which makes it better for weight loss.

High Amount of Dietary Fiber

Fiber is one of the most essential things that help in weight loss. It aids your digestion and regulates your appetite. Natural foods have a lot of fiber in them as compared to processed foods. This makes natural food a great choice for easy weight loss.

Natural Foods Increase Your Eating Time

Food in its natural form is more fibrous and requires more time to eat. You have to chew it more so eating time increases. We know that the longer we take to eat our food, the less inclined we'll get to eat more. Leptin, our satiety hormone will be able to trigger fullness to the brain. This negates the risk of overeating. Whereas, processed food is easy to eat, therefore, you can easily overeat it. It leads to unnecessary piling up of calories.

Real Foods are Packed with Polyphenols

The polyphenol in plant-based foods is a rich source of antioxidants. They help you in fighting inflammation and aid weight loss too. Several flavonoids in the real foods give a real boost to the fat burning hormones and weight loss becomes easy.

No Refined Sugar in Natural Foods

Refined sugar is at the root of this obesity epidemic. Whole natural foods may contain some natural sugar but it is completely harmless; however, they do not contain any refined sugar. This makes natural food best for weight loss.

Refined sugar only adds empty calories and gives way to cravings. The more natural foods you consume the greater are the chances that you'll stay away from cravings.

Zero Artificial Trans Fats

Artificial trans-fat is one of the most dangerous gifts of the processed food industry. It was designed to increase the shelf life of food products and it directly aids weight and belly fat gain. Experiments have shown that animals taking trans-fat gained belly fat much faster. Artificial trans fats also lead to several complications like type 2 diabetes, heart diseases, and other disorders. Natural foods have zero trans-fat; they are completely safe. Processed food, on the other hand, may be sold as zero trans-fat yet the oils used in them develop the negative properties.

Natural Food is Voluminous, Yet Low on Calories

The best thing about natural foods is that you can eat them to your heart's content without worrying about stocking up calories. Natural foods may appear more in quantity but they are low on calories. Whereas, processed foods are rich in added sugar and therefore deliver more calories even in small portions. You will gain weight even by eating small quantities of processed food.

Natural foods are nutritious, healthy, and help in weight loss. They do not add empty calories to your system and require a high metabolic rate to burn them. This makes the right choice for weight loss. If you are really serious about losing weight then ditching processed food should be the way and not counting calories in the food. It isn't the quantity of food but the quality of nutrition that matters more in weight loss.

Chapter 7: Natural Food Plan for Weight Loss

The desperation to lose weight has taken a form of panic. People seem to be in a hurry to lose weight fast and are ready to apply any trick for that. This gives a golden opportunity to the weight loss industry into tricking people to believe that they can lose weight through tricks.

There are some important things to remember if you really want to lose weight.

- Weight loss is very simple. It is not a herculean task. You can effectively reduce weight if you put your heart and mind into it.
- Keep your energy consumption low and try to burn more calories.
- Pay more attention to the quality of food rather than quantity as it is your body that has to process that food later on.
- Do not run behind taste and go for healthy food choices.
- Consuming the macronutrients in a balanced manner is very important. You must choose good food products to obtain the macronutrients.

The 3 Main Macronutrients

Carbohydrates

Go for Unrefined Complex Carbohydrates
Whole grains are the best when it comes to consuming unrefined complex carbohydrates. They are full of fiber and along with energy also provide a lot of essential trace minerals. Neglecting carbohydrates altogether from your diets isn't a healthy long-term policy.

Some food experts categorize carbohydrates as the main evil and the cause of weight problems. This isn't completely true. The source of carbohydrates is the main issue. If you are obtaining your carbohydrates from refined flours, sugar, and other such things, then it is definitely bad. However, carbohydrates obtained from whole grains are not only good but essential too.

Whole grains, starchy vegetables, legumes, fruits, and dairy products provide you with a lot of carbohydrates. Along with carbs, you also get fiber, essential trace minerals, and vitamins. These macro and micronutrients are very important for your health. However, you should remember that carbohydrates are an easy source of energy for your body. Your body likes to run on carbohydrate fuel and as long as it keeps getting a ready carbohydrate supply, it will not switch to burning fat. Therefore, carbohydrate consumption shouldn't be high. You should eat carbohydrates in moderation.

Green leafy vegetables and cruciferous vegetables are an exception here. You can eat them in unlimited quantities. Vegetables are voluminous and offer very few calories. They add a lot of healthy fiber to your gut and are rich in vitamins and minerals. You must eat at least 5-7 cups of vegetables daily.

Whole fruits are also great. They carry lots of vitamins and mineral essential for your health. A nutrient-deprived body can never be a healthy body. You would need the right mix of vitamins and minerals from the natural sources and fruits are great for that. They are sweet and tasty. They make the food delicious. They help you stay away from artificial sweeteners and do not cause cravings.

Dairy products are also essential and they also provide vitamins and minerals. You can consume dairy products in moderate quantities.

Protein

Protein is essential for your growth. Weight loss can also cause muscle loss as the body starts eating muscles first when the energy stores are exhausted. Protein intake is essential to make up for the loss of muscle mass. You can eat plant-based and animal-based protein. Both are good for you and have their positive effects.

Animal proteins are the superior source of protein. Fish, poultry white meat, and lean meats are the best when it comes to animal protein.

Fish

Wild-caught saltwater fishes like salmon, sardine, herring, mackerel, and trout are some of the best fishes to eat. They are full of protein and omega-3 fatty acids. They provide you with a lot of protein and also help in weight loss. However, you can also go for other fishes and seafood too. Eating fresh fish—not canned—is the best in all circumstances. But if you want to buy canned fishes, go for low salt varieties.

Poultry

White meat is lean and you can eat it freely. Skinless chicken is not only tasty it is healthy too. You get lots of protein and it is easy to cook.

Eggs

Eggs are the best when it comes to weight loss foods. It has lots of protein and fat–the perfectly balanced mix that will ensure optimal growth and weight loss.

Lean Meats

When it comes to red meats, you need to be a little cautious. The danger of overeating is always there. Always remember that proteins must be an important part of your daily diet but eating excess protein would also mean overloading your body with calories.

Plant-Based Proteins

There is no doubt that meat is a comparatively richer source of protein. However, plant-based protein has its own unique advantages. Plant protein obtained from legumes and lentils are packed with phytonutrients and cholesterol-lowering fiber. So, even if you want to stick to a vegetarian diet, you have plenty of options to get a healthy dose of protein.

Fat

Fat has been the favorite food of mankind for centuries. Our bodies favor fat as it is a rich and long-lasting source of energy and that's the reason our body is always so keen on storing energy as visceral fat. Healthy fats are good for your body as they cause the least amount of insulin spike. Eating a fat-rich diet ensures that your body switches faster to burning the fat fuel in your body.

You can get healthy fats from fatty fish, nuts, seeds, fruits like avocados, cheese, eggs, olives, etc.

It is always best to avoid low-quality fats like hydrogenated oils or refined oils. Always try to consume the highest quantity of fats through food and not through oil. Even olive oil in large quantities is not good. When you consume fat-rich foods you also consume other healthy things like fiber which help in digestion.

Fat-rich food keeps you satiated for long and your food intake goes down. Your cravings come to an end and you can live a better and more content life.

There is unlimited material scattered all around regarding the proportions in which you can consume these macronutrients. However, several studies have proven that it is not the quantity of the food you eat that matters in weight loss but its quality. If you are eating rich quality food and feel content about it your weight loss will be more effective.

The key to sustainable weight loss is to eat a balanced diet and feel positive about it. The more stressed you remain about your weight, the slower your weight loss would be.

Chapter 8: Easy Breakfast, Lunch, and Dinner Ideas

Breakfast Recipes

Veggie Frittata

Serves 2

Serving Size: ½ Frittata

Ingredients:

1 carrot, peeled and shredded

½ bell pepper, thinly sliced

½ onion, thinly sliced

5-6 cherry tomatoes, halved

2 kale leaves, destemmed and thinly sliced

5 eggs

Black pepper, freshly ground

Coconut oil for cooking

Cooking Instructions:

- Preheat oven to 350ºF.
- Pour some coconut oil into an 8-9 inch ovenproof pan. Put it over medium heat.
- Once the oil is warm, add all the sliced vegetables into the pan.
- Sauté the vegetables until they are soft and brown.
- While the vegetables are getting cooked, whisk eggs in a separate bowl until frothy. Season freshly ground black pepper.

- Once the vegetables are soft and brown, pour the eggs into the pan slowly.
- Reduce the heat and cook on a medium-low flame for 5-7 minutes.
- Without stirring, cook the eggs until they begin to set in the pan.
- Once done, transfer the pan to your oven and bake for over 10 minutes or by the time you start noticing a golden brown layer on top.
- Take out the pan from the oven and slice it for serving.

Sweet Potato Hash and Eggs

Serves 2

Serving Size: 2 Eggs with Hash

Ingredients:

1 large sweet potato, peeled and shredded

4 large eggs

¼ tsp. onion powder

¼ tsp. garlic powder

½ tsp. sea salt

½ tsp. dried parsley

½ tsp. black pepper, freshly ground

Coconut oil for cooking

Cooking Instructions

- Mix the shredded sweet potato with the spices in a large bowl.
- Add some coconut oil into a large pan and bring it to medium-high heat.
- Add the hash into the pan and toss for a short while.
- Cover the lid and bring the heat to medium.
- Allow the sweet potatoes to cook for 5-7 minutes at the least. Keep stirring to avoid burning.
- Plate the hash on two plates.
- Cook the eggs as per your liking.
- Enjoy a savory breakfast with hash and eggs

Hot Pumpkin Patties

Serves: 8

Serving Size: 2 Patties

Ingredients:

4 cups pumpkin, nicely pureed

½ cup kale, chopped

½ cup almond meal

1 tbsp. sesame seeds

1 tbsp. chia seeds

1 tsp. salt

1 tsp. pepper

1 tsp. crushed red pepper

1 tsp. turmeric

½ tsp. cumin

2 eggs, lightly beaten

Coconut oil for cooking

Cooking Instructions:

- Preheat oven to 350ºF.
- Pour some coconut oil in a large cooking pan and bring it to medium-high heat.
- Add the chopped kale until it gets crispy.
- Take a big bowl and pour the pumpkin puree into it.
- Add the seeds into the bowl along with the ground spices.
- Fold the eggs and cooked kale into the pumpkin mixture.
- Prepare a baking sheet and spray it with non-stick cooking spray.

- Drop heaping tablespoons of pumpkin mixture onto the baking sheet.
- Bake for around half an hour.
- Take out the patties when they get firm and golden brown.
- Serve these delicious patties warm.

Lunch Recipes

Zucchini and Sweet Potato Fritters

Serves: 2

Serving Size: 2 Fritters

Ingredients:

1 cup sweet potato, peeled and shredded

1 cup zucchini, shredded

1 egg, lightly beaten

½ tsp. dried parsley

¼ tsp. cumin

1 tbsp. coconut flour

½ tsp. garlic powder

Sea salt and freshly ground pepper as per taste

Oil for cooking

Cooking Instructions:

- To get perfectly browned fritters, wring out the liquid from the shredded zucchini and let it sit on a paper towel for some time to absorb remaining juices.
- Mix the shredded zucchini with the shredded sweet potato and egg. Mix very well.
- In a separate bowl, mix the coconut flour and the spices. Add this mixture to the zucchini bowl.
- Heat oil in a non-stick pan over medium-high heat.
- Divide your zucchini mix into four equal portions and drop them in the pan.
- Using the spatula, press the zucchini mix lightly not more than half an inch.

- Cook the portions until they get golden crisp. Once ready from one side, flip them over.
- Take them out on a paper towel to absorb extra oil.
- Serve warm.

Aromatic Chicken Bites

Serves 3-4

Serving Size: 6-7 chicken bites

Ingredients:

1 pound chicken, skinless and boneless

¼ cup water

½ cup almond meal

½ tsp. cayenne pepper

½ tsp. paprika

1 tsp. garlic powder

½ tsp. crushed red pepper

½ tsp. chili powder

½ tsp. sea salt

2 tsp. Italian seasoning

Cooking Instructions:

- Preheat oven to 400ºF.
- Prepare a metal baking sheet and coat it with non-stick spray.
- Prepare the almond meal and spice mix in a bowl.
- In a separate bowl, whisk egg and water together.
- Cut the chicken into bite-size pieces.
- Coat each chicken piece into the egg mixture and then drop into the spice mix.

- Repeat the process with all the chicken pieces
- Start laying the spice-coated chicken pieces on the baking sheet.
- Cook pieces for a while on one side and then flip them.
- Bake all the pieces for around half an hour or until they turn crispy and golden brown.
- Serve the delicious chicken bites immediately.

Avocado Salad with Eggs

Serves: 2

Serving Size: 5-6 ounces

Ingredients:

1 avocado, ripe

2 eggs, hardboiled

1 tomato, small

Some cilantro

1 fresh lemon, juiced

Sea salt and pepper to taste

Cooking Instructions:

- Slice the avocado, eggs, tomato, and cilantro into small pieces.
- Mix them in a bowl and add lemon juice, salt, and pepper to the mix.
- Toss them well so that the lemon juice, salt, and pepper get mixed properly.
- Serve on top of salad greens or baby spinach.

Dinner

Caribbean Salmon

Serves: 4

Serving Size: 4-6 ounces of Salmon

Ingredients:

2 pounds of salmon fillets

1 garlic clove, minced

1 tsp. sea salt

1 tsp. paprika

½ tsp. black pepper

½ tsp. oregano

½ tsp. cumin

½ tsp. onion powder

½ tsp. chili powder

¼ tsp. thyme

Coconut oil

Mango Salsa

1 ripe mango, diced

1 avocado, diced

¼ cup tomatoes, diced

¼ cup red onion, diced

¼ cup cilantro, diced

1 jalapeno, seeded and diced

½ lime, juiced

Salt to taste

Cooking Instructions:

- Prepare the salsa first. Combine all the ingredients in a bowl and refrigerate them until needed.
- Preheat the grill pan.
- Mix all the spices well in a bowl.
- Properly coat the salmon fillets with the coconut oil, ensuring all sides are coated.
- Rub the spice mix on the fish properly.
- Place the salmon fillets with skin side down on the pan.
- Cover and let them cook for around 3 minutes.
- Cautiously flip the salmon fillets and reduce the heat to the minimum.
- Cover again and cook for about 5 minutes.
- Serve the salmon fillets on the bed of greens and mango salsa on the top.

Chicken Street Tacos

Serves 4

Serving Size: 1 cup

Ingredients:

1 pound boneless chicken

1 head butter lettuce

1 can diced tomatoes

1 onion, diced

1 cup olives, chopped

Cilantro, chopped

Hot sauce

2 tbsp. taco seasoning

Cooking Instructions:

- Place the chicken in a crockpot.
- Add the diced tomatoes along with the taco seasoning to the crockpot.
- Cover the crockpot and cook until it becomes tender and fully cooked. This should take around two hours.
- Take out the chicken. Shred and serve in lettuce wraps. Top it with onion, cilantro, olives, and hot sauce as per your taste.

Chapter 9: Fruits to Make Weight Loss Sustainable

Healthy food is more balanced and lacks artificial sweeteners to add taste to it but it can get boring at times. However, it is very important that you always keep your food interesting or else maintaining it for long would become difficult. Fruits come as a great relief in such circumstances. Fruits add flavor to your food and make it interesting. You have the option to add a lot of fruits to your diet and your weight loss regimen would not remain bland and boring anymore.

Some of the fruits that make your food interesting as well as give you immense weight loss benefits are:

Apple

We have been hearing the age-old saying 'An apple a day keeps the doctor away'. It does have some meaning in it when it comes to weight loss. Apple is a superfruit packed with benefits. The biggest benefit of eating this crunchy and delicious fruit is that it gives you a lot of fiber. They are tasty and it gives you one more reason to eat it. Aside from these, apples are full of antioxidants and phytonutrients too. They help your body in fighting free radicals in your body. Controlled studies have shown that eating apple can lead to substantial weight loss as compared to other whole grains like oats.

Banana

Banana is a nutrient-dense fruit. This potassium-rich fruit can come as your savior when you are having a strong craving to eat sweets. This sweet fruit makes you feel fuller without the disadvantage of loading you with empty calories.
You can eat it in between the meals whenever you feel the urge to snack. It is healthy and nutritious.

Blueberry

Blueberries are rich in water and fiber and an excellent choice on a weight loss regimen. High water and fiber content in this berry helps in lowering the appetite and aids your weight loss efforts. It is rich in antioxidants and helps in fighting the free radicals. So, it not only helps in slimming you down but also provides antioxidant properties.

Grapefruit

This tart fruit is an excellent choice if you want to handle your appetite well. It is full of fiber and eating grapefruit in its natural form helps in keeping your hunger at bay. You also get a lot of water and fiber through this tart fruit.

Pear

If controlling food cravings and keeping your appetite under check is a challenge for you, then you can hit gold with pear. This is a fiber-rich fruit that helps you in keeping your digestion working well. The fiber in pears helps your body in digesting the nutrition from all other foods pretty well. It also helps in controlling your cravings.

Pomegranate Seed

This fruit has amazing health benefits in store as well as weight loss abilities. First of all, pomegranate is loaded with potassium. You need a lot of potassium on a daily basis for healthy living. Eating pomegranate on a regular basis can help you in catering to those needs. Pomegranate is also filled with antioxidants that help in improving your blood flow and decreasing the harmful low-density lipoprotein (LDL) levels. The biggest weight loss benefit of pomegranate lies in its ability to boost your metabolism. High amounts of polyphenols and antioxidants help in better metabolism and you are able to burn calories more effectively. This sweet fruit also helps in regulating your appetite. You must consider keeping this fruit in your food plan.

Orange

This citrus fruit is one of the best when it comes to weight loss. If you want to give your metabolism a kick start then eating oranges is the best strategy. Oranges are filled with thiamine, vitamin C, and folate. They boost your metabolism and increase your calorie-burning abilities. If you are troubled with cravings for food, or if you love the sweet and tangy flavor, then oranges are also great for you.

As a word of caution, stick to eating the fruit in place of drinking them as juice. The pulp and the fiber are the most helpful for your body, so no point in wasting it.

Kiwi

It is a superfood and excellent for weight loss. It is full of insoluble fiber that helps your digestion a lot. It also contains a lot of soluble fiber that also helps you in feeling full for longer. This tangy, sweet fruit is filled with nutrition.

Papaya

Papaya is the perfect fruit for weight loss as it contains an enzyme called papain that helps your digestion system. It is also filled with antioxidants, flavonoids, and vitamin C that add great benefits to your health. You must consider it in your daily fruit intake.

Guava

It is an important fruit even for those who cannot eat sweet fruits due to diabetes. Guava is low on the glycemic index and therefore even the people suffering from diabetes can eat it. It is rich in fiber and greatly helps your digestion. If constipation troubles you a lot, guava is the answer to your problems. The fiber content of guava boosts your metabolism and helps in weight loss.

Chapter 10: Ensure Fat Burn and Prevent Muscle Loss by Eating Right

If you want to lose weight and maintain it in long-term, then you'll have to do more than making some adjustments. Sustainable weight loss requires healthy changes in your lifestyle. Weight loss can only be sustainable if you follow these things as a part of your lifestyle. Quick tricks don't work in this area. Most of the lifestyle changes required are simple healthy habits. They would neither require much of your time or effort. You simply need to follow them mindfully. You'll witness that losing and maintaining weight was never so easier.

Important Things to Follow

Eat Adequate Amounts of Protein Daily

When your body starts catabolism or the process of eating itself to reduce weight it simply doesn't cut fat, there is a substantial loss of muscle mass too. It is an inevitable thing but not dangerous if you are ready to supplement the lost muscles with adequate protein intake.

You must eat a minimum of 56 grams of protein for men and 46 grams of protein for women. You can easily eat this much protein without stressing on anything. A small serving of meat about the size of your palm has much more protein than that.

You should focus on eating high-quality protein. Fish, eggs, lean meat, poultry, lentils, tofu, and dairy–all have the required protein. The important thing is never to miss the daily dose of protein.

Eat Lots and Lots of Fruits and Vegetables

Fruits and vegetables are your best partners when it comes to weight loss. They are low on calories and high on fiber, mineral, vitamins, and nutrients. They also help you in keeping hunger and cravings at bay. They make you feel fuller and more satisfied without stuffing you with extra calories.

Remember healthy weight loss is not only about reducing your calorie intake but also about feeling good and satisfied. If your fruit and vegetable intake is high, you will never feel as if you are starving yourself for losing some weight. This feeling of satisfaction will help you a lot more in weight loss than some calorie deprivation technique.

Reduce Your Carbohydrate Intake

Carbohydrates supply easy energy to your body. They are the main fuel source for your system. However, high intake of carbohydrate diet can hamper your weight loss efforts. A delicate balance should be followed here. You should avoid eating refined carbs and switch to unrefined complex carbs like whole grains. They are slow to digest and lower the risk of excess calorie intake. Completely avoiding carbs can be tough as your food choices get overly limited. Whole grain carb diet also contains some important trace minerals. So, eat carbs in moderation and stay away from refined carbs.

Do Cardio Exercises

Cardio exercises are the best when it comes to burning calories and maintaining lean muscle mass.

You should aim for at least 150 minutes of cardio every week. Performing cardio at medium intensity helps in increasing heart rate and breathing. However, do not overstress yourself.

Walking or running, riding a bicycle, swimming, or dancing are good cardio exercises.

Weight Training

The best way to maintain muscle mass and build lean muscle mass is to engage in weight training.

Weight training or strength training should only be done for 20-30 minutes at a stretch.

You should try to work on every major muscle during each training.

Activities like weight lifting, isothermic exercises, yoga, and pilates are good for you.

You should start weight training with low weights and then increase the weight with each repetition. Beginning the routine with heavy weights can lead to injuries.

Practice weight training at least at an interval of one day. This will give your muscles time to recover.

Get Proper Sleep

Sleep is very important when it comes to weight loss. Lack of sleep can lead to stress and your weight loss may come to a halt. Adequate sleep time also ensures the optimum release of HGH which is a major fat burning hormone.

Lack of sleep impacts your health and weight loss negatively.

Following a healthy lifestyle and eating regimen will ensure that you lose weight at a steady rate and maintain it. It is a long-term measure and ensures that you not only lose weight but also remain happy and content.

If you will follow a healthy lifestyle you will lose weight and also gain lean muscle mass. However, the focus of your life shouldn't only be losing weight and remaining happy. Try to find happiness in any way you can. The happier and content you remain, the easier it will be for you to lose weight and remain fit.

Conclusion

Thank you for making it through to the end of this book. Let us hope it was informative and able to provide you with all of the tools you need to achieve your weight loss goals.

Excess weight is an issue but it isn't something that you can't handle without panic. Reducing weight under stress and burden will be difficult. Weight loss under fad diets and strict food plans do not fetch the desired results.

These are the most important things that you need to understand before you begin your weight loss journey.

Fighting your food is not the right way to lose weight. This book has tried to explain this very simple fact. If you want to effectively lose weight and maintain it for a longer term, then it can only happen by making the right food choices. Weight loss is a comprehensive process. You will need to bring your act together. Sustained weight loss will require a positive change in lifestyle and eating habits.

This book has tried to show that it isn't difficult. You can make a positive change in your food choices easily and that will have a major impact on your weight.

Selecting the right kind of food items is more important than being overly cautious about the number of calories you eat. Calorie-restrictive diets cannot have a long-term impact on your weight. If you want to bring your weight down, you will have to learn to understand and accept the qualities of the food you eat.

This book throws light on the healthy food items that should be included in a weight loss diet. It also explains the ways in which the right foods will affect your excess weight.

Most people have been fighting the weight loss battle on the wrong front. They have spent a lot of time counting calories and fat whereas the real culprit was processed food and refined sugars. This book explains the ways in which refined sugar increases your weight and derails your weight loss plans. If you have to win against the weight issues, then you should be watching the empty calories you dump in your system through them.

The main aim of this book is to make you aware of the real cause of the obesity issue and the ways to counter it.

You can achieve your weight loss aims very well if you follow a healthy diet and stay as close to nature as possible. The more you embrace nature in your food the better your weight control would be. In the end, you must remember that you cannot win by acting against your body. Starving it is not the right way to become healthy. If you really want to get fit, then you will have to get back to healthy eating and rest of the things would fall into place on their own.

Finally, if you found this book useful in any way, a review on Amazon is always appreciated!

BONUS:

** Remember to use your link to claim your 3 FREE Cookbooks on Health, Fitness & Dieting Instantly

https://bit.ly/2EFv31x

Printed in Great Britain
by Amazon